I0423166

Prologue:

Diabetes is now an epidemic in our country. This book offers a plan of action for those with either pre-diabetes or diabetes, as well as for those with or other health issues who want to maintain or regain their health.

The steps offered here will not only help you prevent diabetes, but other chronic diseases that are fueled by inflammation, such as Alzheimer's, Cancer, and Arthritis. In fact, published research has now shown that Alzheimer's disease could be a third form of Diabetes.

As baby boomers move into middle age, it's more important than ever to take a pro-active stance towards your health so that you can fully enjoy every moment of your life on the planet.

Be pro-active. Know your numbers. Diabetes can be a silent disease. Protect yourself and your loved ones by knowing where you stand.

Stand for health!

Teresa Trower 2011

Table of Contents Page

The Heart of the Matter

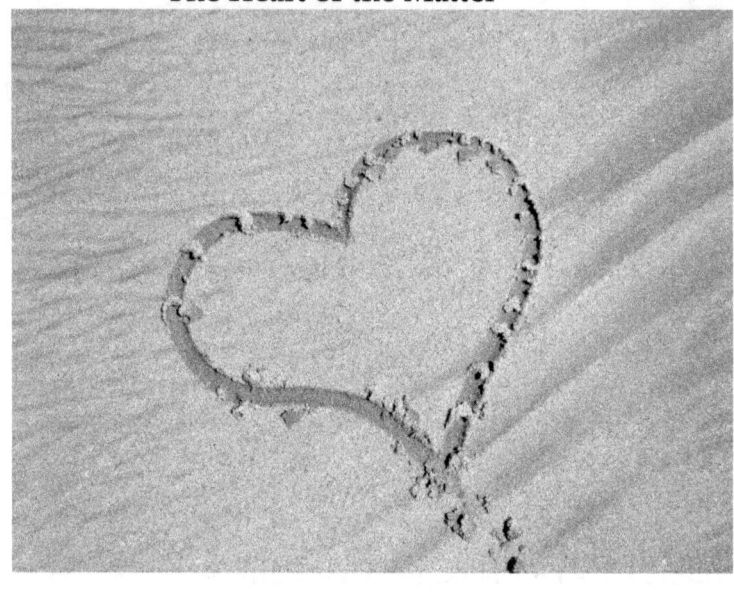

Introduction

As with most people who take up a cause, it was no accident that I was drawn to the topic of Diabetes. Over 30 years ago my mother was diagnosed with Type 2 Diabetes. The diagnosis came from out of the blue. During a routine visit to her opthamologist, she discovered that she had sustained damage to the nerves in her eyes from an excess of sugar in her system. Diagnosis… Type 2 Diabetes. If that was not shocking enough, she was in Stage 4, the most critical.

I witnessed her shock and depression as she realized the many ways in which her life had forever changed. I also witnessed the reality that once diagnosed, the shadow of Diabetes hangs over you for the rest of your life.

My mother lived for only four years following her diagnosis. She was 55 years old.

In 2008, my sister was diagnosed with Type 2 Diabetes. Although she is mindful of keeping herself healthy and following guidelines, managing diabetes will be on her plate for the rest of her life.

My youngest sister, during her first pregnancy, developed what they call "gestational diabetes". This is a diabetic condition that occurs to at-risk women during pregnancy. Although the condition is monitored and usually goes away after pregnancy, it puts her at a higher risk of developing Type 2 Diabetes later in life.

Obviously, heredity is a huge factor. However, there are many controllable factors that will be pointed out in this publication.

I recently read the obituary of a former colleague... cause of death: diabetes. Each day I hear of more and more people who are being diagnosed with not only diabetes, but other chronic diseases as well.

This doesn't have to happen. For this reason, I felt moved to offer some simple guidelines to lower your risk before it's too late. By following the seven simple steps outlined in this book, you can avoid a collision with this, and other life changing diseases. You have the power.

To your health!

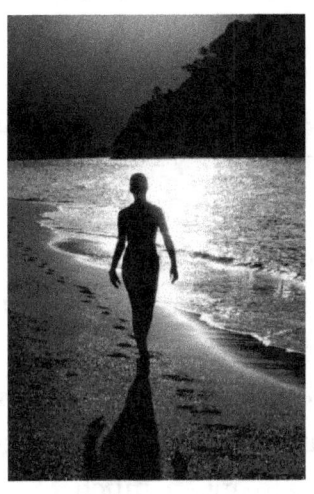

"The journey of a thousand miles begins with a single step."
Lao-Tzu

How To Use This Book

If you have been diagnosed with Pre-Diabetes or have a history of high blood sugar, following the guidelines outlined here will give you the tools to avoid Type 2 Diabetes. If you have a family history, fall into a high risk group, or simply desire to live a healthier lifestyle and avoid chronic diseases, then this is your toolkit to better health.

Step 1, Knowing Your Numbers, comes first because you need to know your blood levels before you can determine your risk level. Before you can benefit from the suggestions laid out in this publication, you need to have your blood work completed and your numbers in hand. The information outlined here is not going to mean much to you if you're unaware of your current levels.

Before you progress to Step 2, have your blood drawn and fill in your numbers. You'll then be equipped with the data to assess your current risk and level and begin to incorporate the suggestions listed in Steps 3-5.

Congratulations for taking the first proactive step towards premium health!

The Good News:

What if you could wake up each day with abundant energy and excellent health? Beyond that, what if your golden years turned out to be some of the best years of your life?

Hard to imagine?

Aren't we programmed with the expectation that our bodies are destined to deteriorate with each passing year beyond the age of thirty? What if we've been sold a belief that actually encourages the very deterioration that we fear?

Research has now demonstrated that chronic diseases such as Diabetes, Cancer, Alzheimer's and Arthritis have definite links to lifestyle and can be prevented and managed by positive changes in lifestyle.

You can take charge of your health. You don't have to anticipate a life of physical decline. Although you can't alter your genetic makeup, by utilizing these simple strategies, you can significantly increase your chances of avoiding the severe side effects of chronic disease and lose unwanted pounds.

The focus of this writing is Diabetes prevention, but these measures can be applied to other chronic diseases as well. You will discover not only where you are now as far as your current risk for disease, but how to move in the direction of more abundant health and vitality.

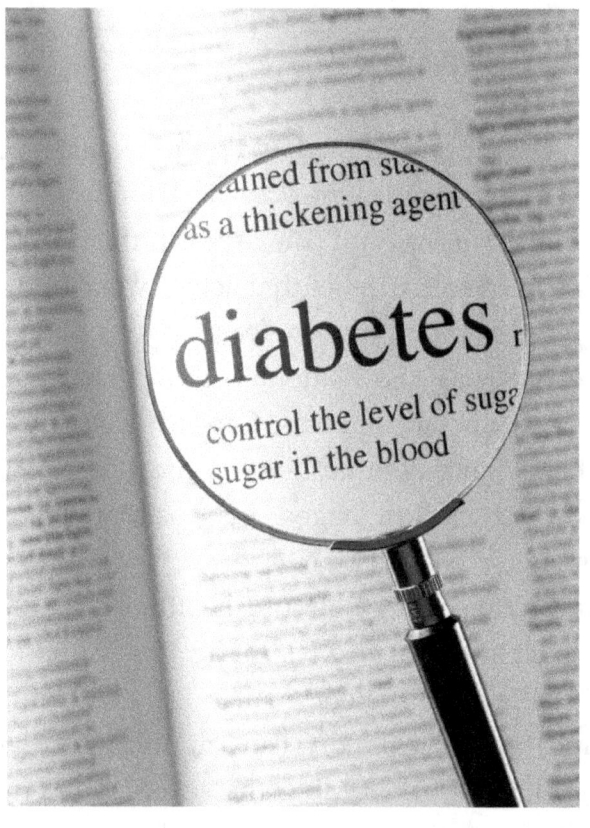

Don't Look Behind You: Diabetes is Catching Up Fast

Why has the incidence of Type 2 Diabetes been steadily increasing in the United States? According to the Center for Disease Control (CDC), nearly 26 million Americans in 2011 suffer from diabetes and an estimated 79 million adults have pre-diabetes. This is a frightening statistic.

What might be contributing to this rising epidemic?

Family history is a major risk factor. Approximately 75% of children with type 2 diabetes have a parent or sibling with the condition. In fact, a family history of Type 2 Diabetes is one of the strongest risk factors for getting the disease. However, it only seems to affect people living a Western lifestyle.

Another risk is ethnicity. African Americans, Asians, Hispanics, and Native Americans are at higher risk.

Age is another risk factor, if you are over 45. A sedentary lifestyle is also a risk, as is having an apple as opposed to a pear shaped torso. Of course, these are the factors that you can't control.

Let's look at the factors that you can control.

Often the propensity for Diabetes is triggered by poor nutrition habits which are learned in the home. The old admonition, "That's not how my mother fixed it," dies hard. Today an estimated 66 percent of adults are either overweight or obese, a major risk factor for diabetes. Fast food meals are still a popular meal replacement for people on the go. Meals around the dinner table are still in a state of decline.

How about stress? Are we more stressed than ever before? My grandparents often knew what was happening in their neck of the woods, but they didn't lie awake at night worrying about how they were going to be affected by the tsunami that occurred somewhere thousands of miles away. Too much stress over-stimulates our delicate autonomic nervous systems and wreaks havoc with the body's nutritional balance.

Although lifestyle is a controllable variable, many today are making poor lifestyle decisions.

In fact, poor nutrition and physical inactivity have replaced cigarette use as the leading preventable causes of premature death in the US.

The good news is that people are beginning to take notice. Physicians are monitoring blood sugar levels and encouraging their patients to make lifestyle changes.

News about the increasing prevalence of diabetes is more often appearing in the media. Articles warning about how the rising costs of treating diabetes continue to appear.

Households with a member with diabetes spend somewhere between 10 to 20 percent of their income on health care. For example, in 2007 the total annual healthcare costs for a person with diabetes was almost $12,000 a year, or $1,000 a month. Do you have an extra $1,000 a month to spend on diabetes? What if you could take that same $1,000 and put it into a savings account? At the end of 5 years, you'd have more than $6,200 saved. This is the financial benefit of avoiding diabetes. Think about it. If you're diagnosed with diabetes at age 45 and you live until 75, that's a lot of moolah going out the door.

Others with different insurance plans, such as flexible spending accounts, report lower costs. Still, diabetes is an expensive disease. Then there are additional costs, including visits to podiatrists, ophthalmologists, and lost wages due to sick days or hospital visits.

For those who are over 65, there is a gap in medical coverage called the doughnut hole. This is a period when Medicare will not pay and the patient is required to cover all medical expenses up to a certain limit. A person using insulin along with other diabetes medications would likely spend over $300 a month on medication and syringes.

Further, persons with diabetes have more difficulty qualifying for health insurance. One study found that 80 percent of people with diabetes were unable to qualify for new health insurance after a job change, a layoff, a move, or a divorce. Also, people with diabetes are less likely to leave a job they dislike because of the real possibility of losing their health benefits.

So, you can see that avoiding a diagnosis of diabetes has huge financial implications. Each day that you're not spending money on health expenses, you're saving that amount for yourself... saving that money for your personal goals.

This book will examine the causes of Diabetes and ways to determine where you fit on the diabetic risk factor scale. By assessing your risk level, knowing your numbers, and tweaking your lifestyle, you can bypass this devastating disease and take charge of both your health and your future.

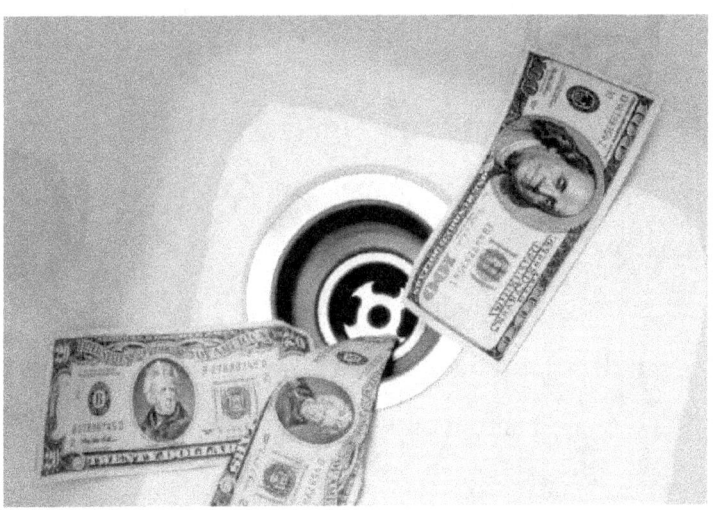

Health Costs... Your Moolah

My Risk Assessment

1. **My motivation for reading this book is because:**

    a) __diabetes runs in my family.

    b) __I know someone with diabetes.

    c) __I have pre-diabetes.

    d) __I have Type I or Type 2 diabetes.

    e) __I want to prevent diabetes.

2. **I have the following risk factors for diabetes:**

    a) __It runs in my family

    b) __I am Afro-American, Asian, Hispanic,
    or   Native American.

    c) __I am overweight.

    d) __I am over 45 years of age.

    e) __I carry weight around the middle.

If you have identified even one risk factor, following the seven steps outlined in this book will help you prevent this disease.

Further, the lifestyle changes prescribed will reduce inflammation, promote weight loss, and improve your immune system's ability to fight disease.

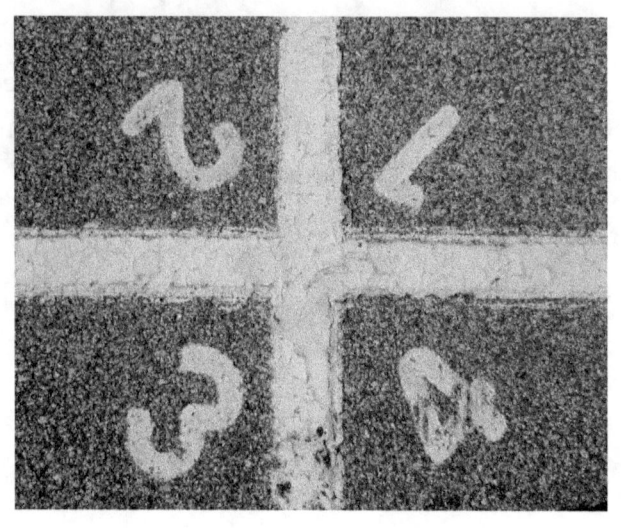

Step 1: Know Your Numbers

Okay, we all know that diabetes is mostly caused by obesity, poor diet, family history, and lack of exercise. But how many of us are a little overweight, eat fast food on occasion, fail to exercise at least three times a week, and feel stressed? I would venture that a majority of Americans fall into this category. So, how to know if you are in the danger zone?

Your body can give you signals that you are on the wrong path. If you find that you are gaining weight around the middle, this leads to inflammation and glycemic stress.

Do you crave sugar? People who are sugar sensitive generally crave sweets, bread, cereal, and pasta, all of which spike blood sugar levels.

You may also have low serotonin levels, suffer from depression, or use alcohol to self- medicate. Many times alcoholism is found in families with sugar sensitivity. People with sugar sensitivities have problems metabolizing carbohydrates and have a different insulin response than those who are not sensitive to sugar.

Depressed yet? The good news, however, is that this condition can be completely reversed! The proof is in the numbers.

How powerful is knowing your numbers? By knowing your numbers and determining your risk, you are in a position to take charge of your health, modify your diet and lifestyle, lower your numbers, and avoid a Type 2 diagnosis completely. Instead of paying for a lifetime of medications, you can spend the money you save on something that empowers you and gives you pleasure.

You may be thinking that you're feeling healthy and fit, and that these statistics don't apply to you. Yet, many people are blindsided when they go in for a regular checkup with their eye doctor only to find out that they have irreversible damage to their eyes from undiagnosed Diabetes. Don't be one of these people. Know your numbers!

There are basically three stages that the body goes through prior to receiving a diagnosis of Type 2 Diabetes. These are Inflammation, or Glycemic Stress, Insulin Resistance, and Metabolic Syndrome.

To know whether you fit into one of these categories, you will need to know your numbers, which can only be determined from a blood test.

The purpose of this book is not to dwell on the dangers of Diabetes, which include blindness, amputation, stroke, kidney disease, and nerve damage, to name a few. Instead, it is to give you tools for prevention. It's never too late to take charge of your health. Your grandchildren deserve to know you!

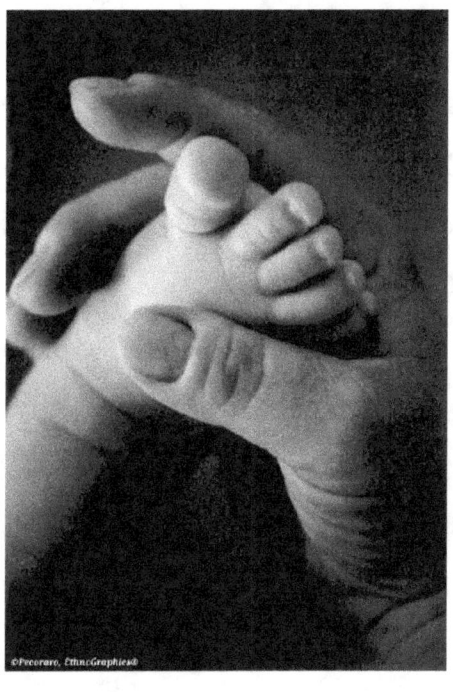

Know Your Numbers

(The following blood levels can be determined through a blood test ordered by your physician.)

What is your most current measurement of:

My Current Numbers	Normal
_____waist size	*<35(F), <40(M)*
_____CRP (C Reactive Protein)	*<3.1*
_____Total Cholesterol	*<200 mg/d*
_____ LDL Cholesterol	*<130*
_____ HDL Cholesterol	*>40 mg/dL*
_____ Triglyceride	*<150 mg/dL*
_____ HbA1c	*<6%*
_____Glucose	*65-99 mg/dL*
_____Vitamin D	*30-100 mg/dL*
_____ Blood Pressure	*<120/*

"Ignorance is not bliss."
Unknown

Step 2: Understand Your Numbers

Waist Size

Your waist size is an important gauge because weight around the middle increases inflammation, which is the first stage leading to Diabetes.

For women, your waist size should be no more than 35", and 40" for men.

To measure your waist circumference, use a tape measure. Start at the top of the hip bone. Pull it all the way around level with your navel. Make sure it's not too tight and that it is parallel with the floor. Don't hold your breath while measuring it!

If your waist size is much higher than the recommended measurements and you feel hopeless to ever attain those numbers, take heart. It is do-able through lifestyle change. But we'll get to that later.

So, how do you know how much inflammation you have in your body and why should you care?

C-Reactive Protein

C Reactive Protein is actually the measure of inflammation in your body. This is an indication of how many white blood cells are being released into your system to fight what your system sees as a foreign invader.

Increased CRP levels have been found in people with type 2 diabetes, gestational diabetes, and metabolic syndrome. Obesity has also been associated with these conditions.

Recent studies have shown that inflammation is a very accurate predictor of future heart problems, another side effect of Diabetes.

If that were not scary enough, elevated levels of C Reactive protein may also double your risk of a stroke.

By the simple process of checking your CRP levels, you can assure yourself that inflammation is not running rampant in your body.

If it is, you can take action by following the steps outlined in this book.

The good news:

You can decrease the level of inflammation in your body through diet, nutrition, and stress management. Just knowing this fact alone should lower your stress!

Total Cholesterol

Cholesterol has been often demonized in the media. But cholesterol, by itself, is not a bad thing. In fact, it promotes positive functions in the body.

Cholesterol is a soft waxy substance found in your bloodstream and your cells and is used in the function of vitamin D, hormones, and cell membranes. I don't know about you, but I want the membranes around my cells to stay strong and provide a sufficient boundary.

However, when your body produces too much cholesterol, it endangers your cardiovascular system….your ticker. So, keeping your cholesterol levels in balance is a life- saving exercise.

Doctors usually recommend that your total cholesterol be below 200. Anything above 240 is considered high. The screening test is called a lipoprotein profile.

What does this mean to you?

High cholesterol is a predictor of diabetes. Elevated cholesterol levels are often seen in people with insulin resistance, even before they have developed full blown Diabetes. Therefore, a link exists between high cholesterol, insulin resistance, and Diabetes.

The good news:

It can be prevented, treated, and managed. Are you beginning to see a pattern here?

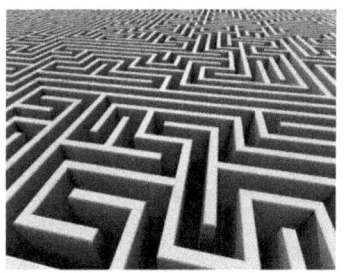

LDL Cholesterol

LDL, or low density lipoprotein, is known as the bad cholesterol. When too much LDL (bad) cholesterol circulates in the blood, it can slowly build up in the inner walls of the arteries that feed the heart and brain.

Together with other substances, it can form plaque, a thick, hard deposit that can narrow the arteries. If a clot forms and blocks a narrowed artery, a heart attack or stroke can result.

A new test is now available which identifies whether your cholesterol consists of large or small particles. Small particles are more dangerous because the big ones are more easily carried away by the flow of blood. This finding may impact your doctor's recommendation and treatment.

Actually, people with diabetes have the same risk for heart disease and stroke as those who already have cardiovascular disease.

The good news:

A person with diabetes who lowers his LDL cholesterol can reduce cardiovascular complications by 20 to 50 percent.

If you haven't been diagnosed with diabetes, you can take preventative action by keeping your LDL level below 130.

HDL Cholesterol

HDL, or high density lipoprotein, is known as the good cholesterol. It is known as "good" cholesterol, because high levels of HDL seem to protect against heart attack. It's thought by medical experts that HDL carries cholesterol away from the arteries and back to the liver, where it's passed from the body. So, as Martha Stewart says, "It's a good thing." If your HDL levels are below 40 mg/dl, however, not much of your bad cholesterol is being transported away.

Triglycerides

Triglycerides are another form of fat manufactured in the body. If you are overweight, rarely exercise, smoke cigarettes, drink alcohol heavily, and eat lots of carbohydrates, this is a recipe for an elevated triglyceride level. Stir in a couple of chocolate bars and you're off the charts!

If you have high triglycerides, you probably also have a high LDL level, which is the bad cholesterol, and a low HDL, which is the good. And you've boarded the Diabetes Express.

The good news:

Triglyceride levels can be controlled with diet. Again, you're in charge. And isn't it better to be in charge? If you could name one person to take control of your cholesterol levels, who would that person be? I hope that your finger is pointing back towards you!

HbA1c

Hemoglobin A1c provides an average of your blood sugar control over a six to twelve week period. A level greater than 5.5% is indicative of pre-diabetes. The advantage of this test is that it shows an indication of your blood sugar over time. Physicians like this!

Vitamin D

Why is Vitamin D important? Vitamin D helps your body utilize the calcium and phosphorus from your food. Vitamin D is probably best known for helping with bone development and the prevention of rickets. Yet, it also prevents cancer by regulating cellular differentiation.

In addition, it helps with insulin secretion, which prevents…guess what… Diabetes.

Why are you more at risk for a Vitamin D deficiency if you are overweight or a vegetarian?

Vitamin D is absorbed by fat cells, so if you are overweight, your vitamin D is being hijacked by your fat cells and you are more likely to be deficient in this important vitamin.

If you are a vegetarian, you may be deficient because many of the foods through which your body attains Vitamin D are animal based, such as eggs yolks, fish, cheese, and some grains.

The good news:

If you are deficient, you can absorb Vitamin D through the skin. Just 10-15 minutes of sun exposure per day can significantly raise your levels. Also, since one of the side effects of low Vitamin D is depression and fatigue, taking a brief walk outdoors can lift both your spirits and your energy levels. It's a win-win.

Taking Vitamin D supplements is another option. Many physicians recognize the importance of Vitamin D for health and prescribe Vitamin D prescription medications for their patients who are deficient. Bottom line...you will feel better when your Vitamin D levels are normalized.

Thyroid

First of all, if your thyroid is malfunctioning, your energy level is affected. If your thyroid is low, you may have no interest in tweaking your lifestyle because you don't have the energy to tweak anything.

Further, your weight gain may be due to a sluggish thyroid and have nothing to do with Diabetes.

However, if your TSH levels are too high, indicating hypothyroidism, this elevates your C Reactive Protein levels, indicating inflammation, a precursor to Diabetes. So, it's always prudent to have your thyroid functioning at full throttle.

The good news:

Your physician can prescribe medications which normalize your thyroid levels. In effect, you'll be lowering your risk level for Diabetes and increasing your energy level and vitality at the same time. It's a win-win!

Blood Pressure:

Have you ever been so angry or stressed that you could actually feel your blood pressure rising? With me, it's somewhat like a tight band of pressure inside my head.

So, what is blood pressure exactly and what causes this uncomfortable sensation? For many people, there are no physical sensations or warnings when their blood pressure is high. Therefore, if you have symptoms, consider yourself lucky.

Blood pressure is the force of blood pushing against the walls of the arteries as the heart pumps blood. If this pressure rises and stays high over time, it can damage the body in many ways.

High blood pressure can cause arteries throughout the body to narrow, limiting blood flow to major organs. It can cause aneurysms, or abnormal bulges, to form in the walls of the arteries. It can also lead to heart failure, kidney failure, or stroke. Bottom line, high blood pressure is nothing to play around with. Your best protection is to avoid it.

You are more likely to develop high blood pressure, or hypertension, if you are overweight or obese.

Other risk factors include drinking too much alcohol, not getting enough potassium in your diet, eating too much salt, not getting enough exercise, and smoking. In addition, having a family history or having chronic stress puts you at higher risk.

If your blood pressure is 140/90 mmHg or higher over time, your doctor will likely diagnose you with HBP. This can be determined by a simple blood test.

To prepare, don't smoke or drink coffee for 30 minutes before the test. Because having a full bladder can affect your blood pressure reading, make sure your bladder is empty. Then, sit quietly for 5 minutes before the test because moving around can raise your blood pressure.

The good news:

You can lower your blood pressure by not smoking, exercising, limiting salt, and following a healthy diet. Medications are also available, but prevention is less costly and just as effective.

Finally, the simple act of knowing your numbers puts you in the driver's seat. There are positive interventions for any problems that you identify, such as high cholesterol or high glucose levels.

However, you can't treat what you don't know exists.

So many people are blindsided when they get a diagnosis of Type 2 Diabetes because they haven't experienced any symptoms.

This is a case where no news is definitely not good news. Knowledge is power. Don't let this chronic disease sneak up on you. Know your numbers!

My Action Plan to Improve My Numbers:

My Numbers	Recommended Activity
Waist size>35"	Exercise and weight loss
C Reactive Protein	Eat more vegetables and less sugar
Total Cholesterol	Avoid red meat and saturated fats
LDL Cholesterol	Take the skin off of the chicken
HDL Cholesterol	Increase my exercise
Triglycerides	Monitor my intake of sugary foods
HbA1c	Implement the seven steps
Glucose	Avoid high glycemic foods (Step 3)
Vitamin D	Get 15 minutes of daily sun before 10 or after 2 o'clock.
Blood Pressure	Lower my stress and frequently check my blood pressure levels

By taking the above recommendations, I can begin to improve my numbers, and therefore improve my health!

Step 3: Conquer Your Cravings

The Glycemic Index

According to Dr. Karen Wolfe, author of *Create the Body Your Soul Desires, The Friendship Solution to Weight, Energy, and Sexuality*, the typical unhealthy breakfast for many folks is a glass of orange juice and a bagel. Sound familiar? Sound healthy? After all, could all of those Florida orange juice commercials be wrong? And isn't a bagel a grain? Aren't grains one of the heroes on the food pyramid? Say it isn't so!

In fact, orange juice is full of sugar. Without balancing it out with a high fiber food, such as steel cut oatmeal, your blood sugar is going to spike.

Your body will then release insulin to bring it back down. Then your body releases cortisol to normalize it back up.

 It's at this point that cravings appear, and if you're sugar sensitive, you know about cravings. When you then satisfy your craving, your blood sugar once again spikes, and you start the entire cycle again.

In order to avoid the cravings (which are usually cravings for sugary foods or carbohydrates), you need to keep your blood sugar levels in a healthy zone...not too high...not too low, or, according to the three bears... "just right".

The glycemic index is actually a measure of how quickly carbohydrates break down into glucose and enter the bloodstream. If the carbs enter the bloodstream too quickly, then your blood sugar spikes. So, this is a case of "slow and steady wins the race".

 Glycemic index tables will show you the exact number associated with your favorite foods.

How do you know which foods are the most healthy if you want to avoid Diabetes and other chronic diseases?

Generally, foods which have a high glycemic index are the foods to minimize. These are any foods with a glycemic index level of 70 or higher. In contrast, low glycemic foods have an index level of 55 or less.

Examples of high index foods are many sweets, white bread, instant white rice, white pasta, white potatoes, white bagels, vanilla wafers, many cereals, and all processed foods.

A good rule of thumb…if it's white, it's probably a high glycemic food that will spike your blood sugar and cause cravings.

Low index foods would include most fruits, vegetables, and low fat proteins…just like your mother taught you.

Although we've been taught to avoid fats, fats have also been given a bad rap. It is actually a good idea to consume the right types of fat with each meal. This is important because the presence of fat slows down the rate of digestion and absorption, which keeps your blood sugar level steady.

Cooking time can also affect the glycemic level of foods. For example, al dente pasta has a lower GI level than longer cooked pasta.

Appropriate fats are the mono-saturated fats, which tend to lower your LDL, or bad cholesterol levels. An example would be olive oil.

Another beneficial fat is an Essential Fatty Acid. This includes both Omega 3's and Omega 6's. Walnuts are an example of a food high in the EFA's. An excellent example of a lifestyle menu incorporating the good fats is the Mediterranean Diet.

On the other hand, the fats to avoid would include the saturated fats, which solidify at room temperature. The unhealthy fats are usually one of the first ingredients listed on the box of a processed food.

Reading the list of ingredients on a box will help you scrutinize whether this product is really something you want to ingest.

The most expedient action you can take, at this point, is to eliminate foods that have a high glycemic index rating.

Remove these items from your pantry. These include cookies, cakes, processed foods, and other foods with a glycemic index level above 70.

Then re-stock the pantry with items such as beans, vegetables, legumes, beef, chicken and vegetable stock.

When you revamp your pantry, you are making a visible commitment to change as well as removing high glycemic foods which spike your blood sugar. Don't underestimate the importance of this step.

How To Know If You're At Risk?

Inflammation is one of the first stages leading to Diabetes. High glycemic foods lead to inflammation and the dreaded free radical formation.

Free radicals can damage the lining of the arteries, not to mention create wrinkles (for the over 40 readers).

Some of the first signs of inflammation, or glycemic stress in your body are cravings, eating at night, gaining weight around the middle, unsuccessful dieting, and afternoon fatigue.

If this sounds like you, take heart. By limiting your intake of high glycemic foods, you can easily reverse this condition. Try listing the glycemic index of everything you eat for a week. This will greatly increase your awareness of the consequences of what you're actually eating.

Untreated inflammation usually moves into a condition called Insulin Resistance. Here it becomes important to have the results of your blood tests, and to know your numbers. Signs of insulin resistance are high triglycerides and low HDL levels.

At this stage, you also experience the carbohydrate cravings that occur when your blood sugar levels are all over the charts.

The final stage preceding an actual diagnosis of Type 2 Diabetes is called Metabolic Syndrome.

At this stage, you not only suffer with the effects from the previous stages, but you now have high blood pressure, with resulting damage to your arteries to add to the mix.

Your fasting blood sugar reading at this stage is 110 or above, and you're now in serious danger of developing Type 2 Diabetes.

Glycemic Index Foods

Here is a list of some high glycemic index foods. These foods have a glycemic index of 70 or higher. For a more complete list of the glycemic index table: http://www.healthyeatingclub.org/info/articles/diseases/glycaemic-table.htm

Generally, high index foods are white, processed, and instant, while low index foods are whole foods such as whole grains, fruits, and vegetables.

Food:	Avg. Glycemic Index
White frozen bagel	72
Whole wheat bread	77
Commercial Cereals	80
White Bread/Rice	70
Rice Cakes	78
Microwave Popcorn	72
White Potatoes	80
Watermelon	72

Five Foods To Avoid For A Longer Life

According to Melanie Haiken, a writer for Caring.com, there are five foods that can trigger a stroke. Therefore, these are the foods that you need to avoid if you want to stay healthy and long in the tooth.

- crackers, chips, and processed foods.

- Smoked and processed meats

- Diet soda

- Red meat

- Canned soup and prepared meals

Processed foods are high in trans fats. She cites the worst offenders as onion rings, French fries, and fried chicken.

The nitrates found in smoked and processed meats, such as pastrami, hot dogs, bacon, or smoked turkey, are not only associated with a higher risk of stroke, but also with a higher risk of Alzheimer's. According to Haiken, nitrates are also associated with a higher risk of leukemia and numerous other types of cancer.

Drinking a soda a day may increase your risk of stroke by 48 percent. In addition, the sugar substitutes in a diet drink are questionable.

Red meat is loaded with artery clogging fat which produces plaques. This plaque buildup is what causes the blockages leading to heart attacks and strokes.

Women are catching up to their male counterparts in the heart attack and stroke category. Since women lose the protective effects of estrogen after menopause, and many women have the potential to live to 100, eating red meat on a daily basis is playing with fire.

Canned soups and prepared foods are found in the middle of the grocery store and require no refrigeration. Their primary means of preservation is through the addition of high amounts of salt, or sodium to the food.

People who consume more than 4,000 mg. of salt double their risk of stroke. Further, salt raises blood pressure, another risk factor for stroke.

Get into the habit of reading the labels to inform yourself of the sodium content, as well as the nitrate and trans fat levels of your food.

Read as if your life depends on it, because in actuality, it does!

My Low Glycemic Plan

Make a list of your favorite foods or snacks. Then list the glycemic index level of that food. Any food with an index level over 70 is considered to be a high index food. Commit to a lower index food to substitute. You don't have to give up your favorite foods, but simply having the awareness that you're eating a high index food can be motivation to make more positive choices.

Favorite Food	Index Rating	Substitution Food

The Inflammation Highway...Fast Lane to Disease

All chronic disease has one thing in common...inflammation. If you suffer from diabetes, arthritis, fibromyalgia, cancer, dementia, or any other long term disease, then you are afflicted with inflammation.

You now know that inflammation is associated with insulin resistance, a stage 2 risk factor for diabetes. So, how does inflammation impact you, and why is it so important to control?

First of all, when your body perceives a threat to its homeostasis, it sends out the white blood cells, your killer cells, to wipe out the threat. You see, your body has your back even when your mind might not!

According to Dr. Mark Hyman, author of *The UltraMind Solution*, inflammation becomes problematic "when your immune system gets confused, and your own tissues get caught in friendly cross-fire. Your body is fighting something... an infection, a toxin, an allergen, a food, or the stress response, and somehow it redirects its hostile attaché on your joints, your brain, your gut, your skin, or sometimes your whole body."

Inflammation in the body creates oxidation. Then, the oxidation creates more inflammation.

One way to think about this is to picture the oxidation process that occurs when you leave half of an apple in the kitchen. The apple turns brown, or a rusty color, as a result of oxidation.

How do you know if you're eaten up with inflammation? To discover your own inflammation level, your doctor can order a blood test for C Reactive Protein, which measures the level of inflammation in your body. How simple is that?

If you do suffer from excess inflammation, there are several ways to lower inflammation. For example, you may be allergic to a certain food, and that can be determined by your physician or through an elimination diet.

You may be going through a particularly stressful time in your life, and engaging in calming activities such as yoga, meditation, and simplifying your schedule can be helpful.

Foods, however, can be part of the problem. Many foods are heavily sprayed with pesticides.

Foods with thin skins absorb the pesticides into the meat of the fruit. Therefore, washing the peel doesn't prevent you from ingesting the pesticide.

The Value of Taking Antioxidants

This is where antioxidants enter the picture. Antioxidant supplements help to neutralize the effects of oxidative stress, or inflammation, on your body.

Many people are not getting enough antioxidants from their food to do the job. Therefore, you can limit the damaging effects of oxidation by taking antioxidants.

As with any supplement, you would be advised to check with your physician before starting a vitamin regimen. The benefits of supplementation are life enhancing and help you maintain your health as well as avoid the chronic diseases that are caused by inflammation.

Antioxidants would include multivitamins, vitamins A,C,D,E, and many minerals, such as selenium, lycopene, and zeanxanthin. Other protective supplements include Chromium, Magnesium, the B Vitamins, Omega 3 Fish Oils, and Grapeseed Extract.

Supplements are better absorbed when taken with food. Taking them at meal time is advisable. In addition, some vitamins need to be taken at different times of the day because the body will only absorb a certain amount at once.

Because the supplement industry is unregulated, meaning that there is no guarantee that what it says on the bottle is actually in the supplement, it is important to take pharmaceutical grade supplements.

Supplements which are pharmaceutical grade meet the same criteria as prescription medications. In other words, what is says on the label is actually what is in the supplement. Vitamins which are not pharmaceutical grade are not held to this high manufacturing standard.
 For example, fish oil supplements can contain mercury, so you have to find the purest forms of fish oil to be safe.

Good sources to check out vitamins would be *Consumer Labs* at ConsumerLabs.com or *The Comparative Guide to Nutritional Supplements* by Lyle McWilliam at Amazon.com.

Cravings:

As previously mentioned, cravings are caused by dips and spikes in your blood sugar levels. The more stable you are able to keep your blood sugar, the fewer cravings you will experience.

Can cravings be caused by emotions? Many people turn to food to calm their racing thoughts or tumultuous feelings. If this sounds like you, take heart. There are actions you can take to calm these emotions. But we'll talk about those later.

Another cause of cravings is adrenal fatigue. When you're feeling exhausted, it's tempting to turn to a sugar or carbohydrate for a quick pick-me-up. The problem is that although the sugar and carbs do give you a temporary boost, what goes up must come down. That surge of energy eventually plunges and you then re-experience the fatigue and the cravings. It's like a rollercoaster ride that you can't get off.

You may feel like a victim of your cravings. Resist the temptation to brow beat yourself for your lack of willpower.

Cravings have nothing to do with willpower and everything to do with your physiology and the food choices you're making. And food choices can be changed.

How To Deal with Cravings:

For some people, sugar is a drug…a powerful drug. As such, it can create addiction. If you find that you have great difficulty staying away from sugary foods, keep a food diary for a week or two to discover how much sugar you're actually eating. You may be surprised. Many foods contain hidden sugars.

Read the labels on everything you eat to educate yourself as to which of your favorite foods contain these hidden sugars.

You may think that you're not taking in sugar, when in actuality you're accumulating sugars through other sources.

Not all sugars are created equal. Some sugars are high on the Glycemic Index level and others are not. Become a wise consumer and use the sugars that aren't going to spike your blood sugar.

Sugars To Avoid:

I don't know about you, but I grew up eating peanut butter sandwiches with peanut butter slathered on white bread. This was the lunchtime staple of my childhood and holds many wonderful memories. Unfortunately, our mothers didn't have the nutritional information we have today, and whole wheat bread wasn't plentifully stocked on the supermarket shelves. Today, however, there are so many healthy breads to choose. Besides, the wheat breads are chewier, have more fiber, and are more filling.

Refined table sugar is another demon on the list. This sugar is commercially processed and stripped of all its beneficial properties. It depletes calcium and magnesium from the bones. It has no nutritional value and is high in calories. Worst of all, it will put weight on you quickly. It's the gift that keeps on giving.

Another high glycemic sugar is high fructose corn syrup. High fructose corn syrup is added to so many processed foods that it's difficult to find a processed food without this ingredient. High fructose corn syrup has been linked to diabetes. Avoid it whenever possible.

Finally, sodas and colas are full of sugar. One soda usually has as many as 10 teaspoons of sugar. Others may have artificial sweeteners, and call themselves diet drinks, but these can be toxic and lead to weight gain.

The Best Alternatives To Sugar:

The sugars found in fruits, called fructose, have a glycemic index level of 19. Fruits are healthy and high in fiber, which has the additional benefit of filling you up…not out!

Stevia has a glycemic rating of less than one. It is 200-300 times sweeter than sugar. If you like the taste, this is an alternative.

Xylitol is a natural sugar sweetener found in the fibers of fruits and vegetables. It is also found in some chewing gums. In fact, my dentist placed this chewing gum in a prominent position at the check-out.

Another choice is Agave Nectar, which is made from the Blue Agave plant. It has a pleasant taste and won't spike your blood sugar. It gets an "A". These sugars can be found in natural food stores and are beginning to be carried in most traditional food chains.

So, now it's time for a reality check...I know you love sugar. I know you have no intention of completely banishing table sugar from your life. Sugar is everywhere. It's hard to avoid it even if you are reading labels. However, if you care about your health, and you want to lose weight and eliminate cravings, you must curtail your sugar intake and avoid high glycemic foods. You can do this! It's about moderation, not starvation.

The Plan:

To curb your cravings, you need a plan. As I quote from Stephen Glenn, "If you don't stand for something, you'll fall for anything."

Stand for something. You must decide what your goal is. If your goal is to curb your cravings, announce it. Affirm it. Believe it. Tell the neighbors. Tell your spouse. Get them on your team. These people can be your greatest allies or your greatest saboteurs.

In the book, *Change Anything*, authors Patterson, Grenny, Maxfield , McMillan, and Switzler, examined the science behind what leads to successful change. Interestingly, they found that willpower was not the critical factor. Motivation, however, was extremely important.

Deciding why you want to curb carbs is crucial to your success. It doesn't matter what motivates you as long as it really motivates you. Don't adopt someone else's "should" as your motivation. For example, "I want to curb my cravings so my husband will get off my back about losing weight," is your husband's motivation. Make sure you own it…that it belongs to you.

Here are a few additional suggestions to help tame the cravings beast.

- **Pay attention to when you're the most tempted to give in to cravings**.

  Yes, I know you're going to experience cravings, so that's a given. The important piece is your plan for how you're going to deal with the cravings when they come. Shadow yourself for a week and write down every situation in which you find yourself craving a food.

- **Note where you are, who you're with, what you're doing, and how you're feeling**.

  Devise a Plan B and write it down. For instance, "When I'm at the movies with Ann, I'll bring my own low glycemic bar instead of eating the popcorn."

- **Make a commitment, and follow through**.

  Because you've added Ann to your support team, she's not likely to plead with you to order popcorn. If your husband is on your support team, he's less likely to bring high glycemic sweets into the house to tempt you.

- **Make sure that you're drinking enough water throughout the day**.

  Dehydration can disguise itself as hunger. Sometimes you can derail a craving just by drinking a glass of water.

- **Print out a copy the glycemic index and tape it to your refrigerator**.

  Find out which foods are high and avoid them. If you can't avoid them, limit them. Baby steps are better than no steps at all!

- **Learn to recommit**.

  There will be times when you slip, when you falter, when you give in to temptation. It isn't necessary to go cold turkey. This is your plan. You can design it to fit your lifestyle and your needs. If you falter, pick yourself up and recommit. Tomorrow is another day. You can do this!

- **List your favorite distractions**.

  Distracting yourself when you're feeling a craving is a winning tactic. Sometimes all you need is a fifteen minute distraction to derail the craving. Don't wait until you're craving the food to think of a distraction. Have a list on the counter. Be prepared!

- Write down your eating schedule and make snack packs. You can combine a fruit with a fiber, such as an apple with walnuts or cheese and celery for a healthful and filling snack.

Finally, although fruit doesn't pack quite the punch of sugar, when you start to limit sugar from your system, you'll find that an apple can be pretty sweet. Besides that, it's filling, full of fiber, and one of the healthiest foods on the planet!

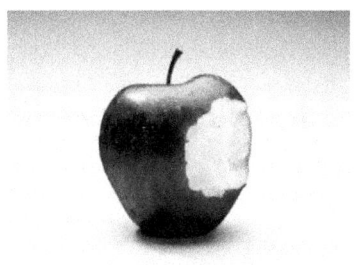

An apple a day....

Remember the old adage, "An apple a day keeps the doctor away.

It's been determined that eating an apple a does more for your brain than previously thought.

Researchers from the University of Massachusetts have discovered that eating an apple can boost your brain power and even help fight off age-related brain damage by maintaining acetylcholine.

Antioxidant-wise, red delicious apples pack the most punch.

- Remember to eat every 3-4 hours. By eating with this frequency, you'll keep your blood sugar steady.

My Plan To Conquer My Cravings

I will implement the following steps to conquer
my cravings:

_____

_____

_____

Antioxidant supplements I would like to add to
my daily vitamins:

_____

_____

_____

The emotions and feelings that are the biggest
triggers for my stress eating are:

_____

_____

_____

Step 4: The Role of Exercise:

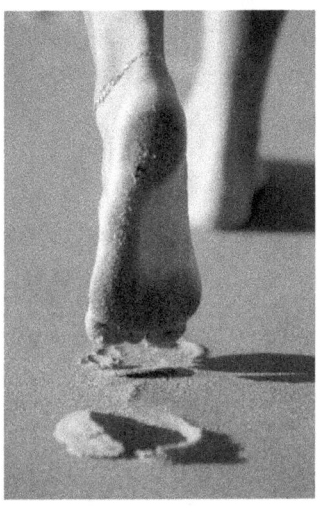

You knew it was coming. We can't talk about health and Diabetes prevention without talking about exercise.

Why? Exercise has a stabilizing effect on blood sugar. It sends sugar away from the bloodstream and into the muscle cells. It reduces cravings.

Blood sugar levels decrease after exercise. This means that there is less glucose in the bloodstream after physical activity, which allows people to manage their glucose more efficiently.

In addition, exercise reduces body fat, which increases the number of insulin receptors. The more insulin receptors an individual has, the greater the sensitivity to the effects of insulin.

Since weight around the waist is a risk factor for Diabetes, using exercise to keep your waist within guidelines is a great prevention tool. The preferred activity level is five or six times a week for 30-60 minutes.

Did I hear a gasp? This may sound like a lot of time devoted to exercise, but if you can find a way to make it into a fun activity, you are more likely to put in the time.

Whether it's walking with a friend, running, doing the elliptical, yoga, aerobics classes, or martial arts, find something that you enjoy and make a commitment for your health.

In fact, just walking for 30 minutes three or four times a week is enough to elevate your metabolism, control your weight, your blood sugar, and your mood.

Woo-hoo!

My Exercise Regimen

Check the descriptions that most closely match you.

__ I never exercise.

__ I make a stab at it, but don't stay with it long.

__ I work out several times a week.

__ I have exercise equipment that I never use.

__ I exercise at home several times a week.

__ I prefer to exercise alone.

__ I prefer to exercise with a group.

__ I get discouraged because I'm in bad shape.

__ I tell myself that I don't have time to exercise.

__ I get bored when exercising. It's torture.

__ I can't afford a gym membership.

__ I am willing to recommit to exercise!

If you indicated that you are even *willing* to recommit to exercise, give yourself a pat on the back. Actually, it doesn't take much exercise to make a difference in your energy level and your muscle tone.

Weight lifting is also a stress reducer. I challenge you...just try it!

If you hate the gym, put your exercise equipment in front of a TV set. Make an exercise corner!

If you don't have room, buy a DVD and walk along with a trainer. These can be found in many chain stores and are reasonably priced.

If you're discouraged because you're not in good shape and it seems hopeless, take baby steps. The latest research survey indicates that it only takes 15 minutes a day to stay in shape.

Remember, the biggest predictor of your weight loss will be your food consumption, so your exercise is a bonus!

I know that you're busy. For this reason, if at all possible, plan your exercise at the beginning of your day. Once your day has started, a million little interruptions, distractions, and unplanned activities can swallow up the time you'd dedicated to exercise.

May people complain that they don't have time to exercise. However, this is a matter of values. What are you valuing more than your health?

Try reminding yourself that exercise may be the most important thing that you've accomplished that day!

What are you willing to commit to?

_____

To whom will you be accountable?

_____

How will you motivate yourself?

_____

How will you reward yourself?

_____

Step 5: Meal Planning

Many studies point to the weight loss success of people who create a food diary. These are the people who take off weight and keep it off.

The" keeping it off" part is where many people fall off the wagon. After going through the initial determination to lose the weight, the weight slowly creeps back on due to attrition. This means, basically, from neglect.

When someone is focusing much of their attention on their goal of losing weight, they pay attention to what they eat. However, as soon as the goal is attained, their attention wanes and they slowly fall back into old, familiar eating routines.

This doesn't have to happen. One way to insure that you will maintain your desired weight is through keeping a meticulous food journal. Keep it in a handy spot in your kitchen and write down everything you eat, including snacks and drinks.

This may not be easy at first, but when you discipline yourself to record your food intake, after about 21 days it will become a habit.

Then it's just another thing on your to-do list, like brushing your teeth, another activity that you do without thinking.

How many days do you skip brushing your teeth because you just "forgot"? Is keeping your desired weight as important as having fresh breath? Think about it...

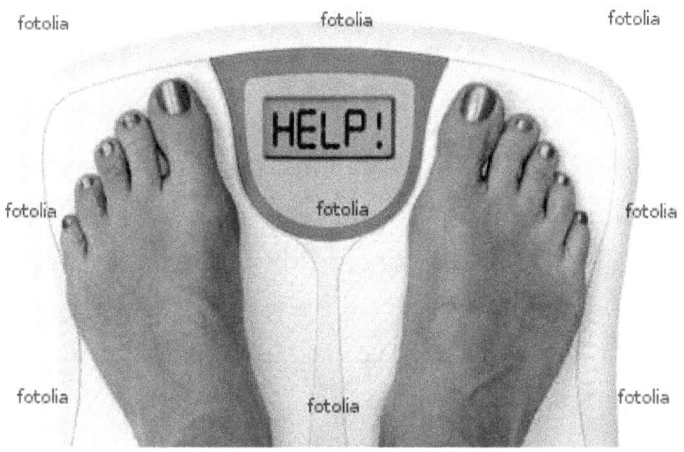

I am what I eat...

A Balanced Meal

What constitutes a balanced meal? The old food pyramid is history. (I always wondered how we could get away with so many grains).

The new food pyramid guidelines recommend that half of your plate be filled with fruits and vegetables.

The other half should consist of a protein and grains. Your protein, which is usually meat, fish, or beans, should be no larger than the palm of your hand.

Now, I realize that this may look like the amazing shrinking protein, but these are the guidelines. There is power in knowing the guidelines, because you can adjust your portion sizing accordingly. At least, you're filling your plate as an informed consumer!

I have just three words for you in making these changes...baby steps, baby steps, baby steps...

Okay....six words.

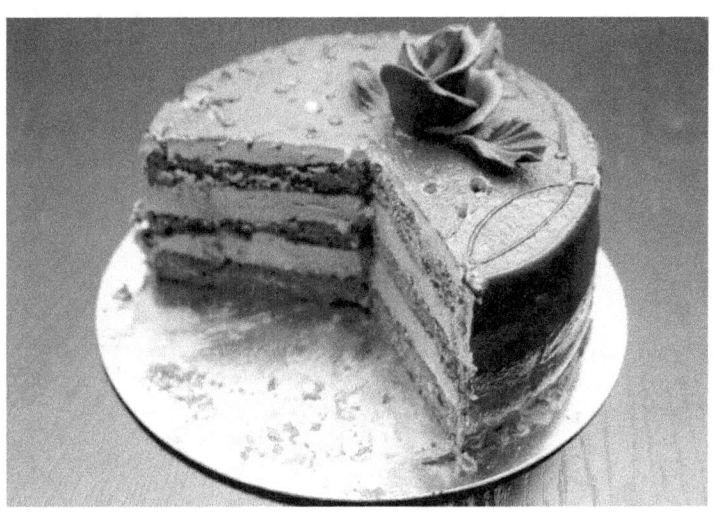

This does not qualify as a balanced meal!

On the following page is an example of a food journal. You may want to design your own. The important thing is to make one and use it!

Food Journal
Week _____

Day	Breakfast	Lunch	Dinner	Snacks

Organic or Non-Organic: This is the Question

In our society today, we are exposed to more toxins than previous generations. We put pesticides on our lawns, in our homes, in our offices, and worst of all, on our foods.

Pesticides are a known carcinogen. The question is…how many toxins can your body fend off before it becomes saturated?

Everyone is different because each person's immune system is operating at a different level.

One of the most positive things you can do to limit your exposure to pesticides is to eat organic. However, organic food is more expensive than non-organic. Maybe you can't afford the extra expense, but you still want to protect yourself and your family.

Not all foods are contaminated by the pesticide treatment. However, in foods with thin skins, the pesticides seep into the meat of the food. Therefore, due to the high concentration of pesticides on those particular foods, it is recommended that you buy those foods only in their organic form.

Foods To Eat Organic

- Strawberries and Blueberries

- Rice

- Bananas

- Baby Food

- Green Beans

- Red Bell Peppers

- Apples

- Peaches

- Cherries

- Grapes

- Soybeans

- Potatoes

- Raisins

- Corn

- Milk … may contain Bovine Growth Hormone

My Weekly Meal Plan

Planning your meals in advance is a tool to keep you from impulse eating. Use the following to plan your evening meal and snacks.

Monday:

Fruit_____

Vegetable:_____

Protein:_____

Grain:_____

Snacks:

(am)_____

(pm) _____

Tuesday:

Fruit_____

Vegetable:_____

Protein:_____

Grain:_____

Snacks:

(am)_____

(pm) _____

Wednesday:

Fruit_____

Vegetable:_____

Protein:_____

Grain:_____

Snacks:

(am)_____

(pm) _____

Thursday:

Fruit_____

Vegetable:_____

Protein:_____

Grain:_____

Snacks:

(am)_____

(pm) _____

Friday:

Fruit_____

Vegetable:_____

Protein:_____

Grain:_____

Snacks:

(am)_____

(pm) _____

Saturday:

Fruit_____

Vegetable:_____

Protein:_____

Grain:_____

Snacks:

(am)_____

(pm) _____

Sunday:

Fruit_____

Vegetable:_____

Protein:_____

Grain:_____

Snacks:

(am)_____

(pm) _____

It is not enough to take steps which may someday lead to a goal; each step must be itself a goal and a step likewise.
Johann Wolfgang von Goethe

Step 6: Master Your Emotions

The Problem with Stress

Stress kills. That's the problem in a nutshell. Stress can annihilate your immune system to the point that, instead of defending your cells against invaders like cancer or inflammation, it responds with barely a whimper.

Is this the wimpy response that you want from your one and only immune system? Really?

Isn't everybody stressed these days?

Everyone does experience a certain degree of stress because life, by its very nature, is full of challenges, worries, and obstacles.

However, not everyone experiences stress on a daily or ongoing basis.

The body is designed to cope with the ravages of stress for brief, or acute periods. It is when the stress becomes ongoing, or chronic, that the effects on the body can become damaging.

How does this happen?

When you perceive a threatening situation, which can be activated by a conscious or unconscious trigger, your body immediately responds by releasing a cascade of chemicals. It's as if the General has called out the Cavalry.

Basically, your autonomic nervous system has two divisions, the sympathetic and the parasympathetic.

You can think of the sympathetic nervous system as the gas pedal, which provides the energetic juice to respond to the threat.

The parasympathetic, which is more like the brake pedal, turns off the juice and restores you to a sense of calm.

If you're constantly revving your car engine, you'll eventually flood the engine and render it useless.

Similarly, if you're constantly putting your sympathetic nervous system in the "on" position, you'll unwittingly set up a chain of potentially negative reactions.

The Effects of Cortisol:

When your sympathetic nervous system is activated, it releases the stress hormone called cortisol. Cortisol, which is made by the adrenal glands, suppresses the immune cells ability to activate telomerase, a cell enzyme that keeps cells young.

Translation: cortisol in this corner...fountain of youth in this corner!

Aside from premature aging, when your adrenal glands become fatigued from releasing too much cortisol, you can also experience fatigue.

Another damaging side effect of cortisol is seen in its effect on the good prostaglandins. Prostaglandins are hormone-like cellular messengers which are derived from essential fatty acids. They're important in decreasing inflammation and boosting your immune system. These protective functions are hampered when you have too much cortisol coursing through your body.

So, let's see. Cortisol can hamper both your good looks and your immune system...not exactly the hormone you want to invite for dinner.

By the time you realize you're stressed, the process is well under way. Your face may be flushed, your breathing shallow, your muscles tense, your heartbeat racing, your hands and feet cold, your digestive system running amok, and your sweat glands pouring. At this point, you not only feel stressed…you look stressed!

The good news:

You can take your foot off the gas and turn off the sympathetic nervous system by doing what you do naturally … by breathing.

When you take a deep, diaphragmatic breath, this action has the power to turn off the sympathetic nervous system, or stress response, and turn on the calming parasympathetic nervous system.

Most people, however, breathe in a shallow manner from the chest. After all, haven't we all been taught to sit up straight and suck in our stomachs? …great for posture…bad for stress. In fact, try taking a deep breath from the belly while holding in your stomach. Impossible!

Diaphragmatic breathing is easier to learn if you are lying on a flat surface on your back. If you place your hand upon your belly button and visualize your belly as a big balloon, you can more easily allow your belly to expand with air.

When you breathe from your belly, you can feel the difference. This type of breathing is extremely relaxing. When you become proficient at this type of breathing, try it standing up. Soon, you'll be able to do the diaphragmatic breathing no matter where you are or what you are doing.

If your anxiety takes the form of a panic attack, you'll need to practice this skill, as well as distract yourself by moving into a different room, if possible.

Although breathing alone may not stop a panic attack, it can minimize the discomfort. Don't take the healing power of your breath for granted! The breath is a powerful weapon against stress, and it doesn't cost a dime.

There are other efficient ways to manage stress…something as simple as listening to music or getting a massage can be an instant stress reducer.

Music has a powerful effect on the emotions and the immune system.

Yoga is also an effective stress reducer. My experience of yoga is that I usually begin the session with a certain degree of tension built up from the day and leave feeling like a wet noodle.

Starting a regular yoga practice, even if you practice only 15 minutes a day, can have a calming effect that carries you through the rest of the day.

Finally, meditation calms both the mind and body. Meditation means being so deeply absorbed in one thought or activity that your mind tunes out everything else.

Some people meditate by focusing on their breath.

Others find spiritual readings or a certain word that resonates a feeling of peace. Then they focus on that, gently pushing away any intrusive thoughts.

Trust me…this can be a mental challenge. Have you ever tried focusing on just one thing for longer than a minute?

This is why they call it a discipline, and call meditation a practice. However, the practice results in increased peace of mind and mental focus, especially when continued over time.

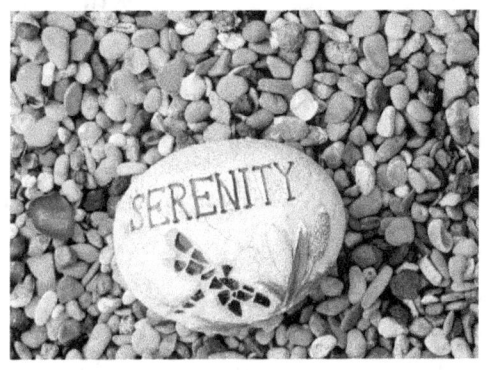

Your greatest ally in the road to health!

Depression, Anxiety, Stress...Oh, My!

According to studies by Knol, et al in 2006, depression increases the risk for type 2 diabetes by 37%. In a series of studies involving over 6,000 cases, the risk for diabetes was 60% higher for those who were suffering from depression.

In fact, middle aged women who experienced depression, stress, tension, and frequent anger were found to be more likely to develop metabolic syndrome.

For men, only one or two stressful life events was all it took to increase their risk for Diabetes.

Interestingly, anger, which is associated with both anxiety and depression, was most highly correlated with the onset of Type 2 Diabetes regardless of gender. Cynicism, in particular, seemed to be the factor most associated with impaired glucose.

The role of work stress has also been implicated in several studies as a causative factor.

Female workers who had experienced tension on the job for at least five years were more likely to develop Diabetes. Burnout has also been cited as a risk factor, but this seems to only affect women.

Emotional worry that interferes with getting at least seven hours of sleep also elevates your risk. Difficulty in maintaining sleep is associated with an 84% higher risk of developing Diabetes. Since untreated depression affects the quality of sleep, it is yet another factor that increases your risk for developing Diabetes.

Before you get depressed from hearing this information, just remember that knowledge is power, and you can use this knowledge to tweak your lifestyle and make powerful changes! So there!

Behavioral Risks

When you're under a great deal of stress, are you feeling and acting at the top of you game? This is more likely the time when gravitate toward both the fast food line and the couch. Exercise is probably not on your radar screen. Even the simplest task may seem like a giant endeavor.

If you're a smoker, you may find yourself reaching for more cigarettes than usual. If you tend to use alcohol to calm your nerves, you may tend to over-imbibe.

None of these behaviors are helpful, at best, and at worst, put you at increased risk of developing Diabetes.

The good news:

Although multiple studies have drawn a link between depression and diabetes, there are actions you can take to diminish your risk. When you're feeling stressed or depressed, it is critical that you pay attention to your feelings. Don't be like the frog that slowly boils to death in the boiling pot.

If necessary, rate your happiness each day on a scale from 1-10. Notice when your happiness or serenity is being challenged or beginning to slip.

Simply going through the ritual of filling out a survey of your mood could be one of the most effective preventive measures you can take on a daily basis.

When you pay attention to your happiness level, you begin to value your happiness more.

Then, when your happiness levels begin to nosedive, it becomes a red flag indicating that something needs to change.

Are you working too hard, worrying too much, or sleeping too much or too little? Is your life out of balance? Are your relationships out of sync and unsatisfying? You get the picture.

Knowing where your dissatisfaction lies is a pointer to the solution. Change is usually called for in some area of your life.

Identify the changes that you desire and decide which changes are within your control. Even those changes that are not within your control can be tweaked.

For example, if job stress is an issue, is there a small change that you can implement? If not, can you reframe your attitude toward the issue and see it from a different perspective.

What small actions could you take to make the situation less stressful? What actions could you take outside of work to lower your stress level? Baby steps can be huge!

The main focus here is to be self-diagnostic as far as your own happiness is concerned. Then, be proactive in implementing change, no matter how small.

Some people develop more serious conditions, such as major depression or anxiety disorders. This is different from the stress that most people experience as a normal part of living.

Major life challenges or genetic predisposition to anxiety or depression can send you into a tailspin of emotion.

If this is you, take heart. These are treatable conditions when supervised by a licensed physician and /or therapist.

When these conditions are managed, they are no longer risk factors for Diabetes.

My Stressbuster Plan

The following activity will help you identify the areas of your life that are most stressful and those that are most rewarding. Look at each area listed below and decide how satisfied you are with this particular area of your life.

1= Not satisfied at all   2= Somewhat satisfied   3= Very Satisfied

__ Fun and Recreation

__ Work and Career

__ Social Relationships

__ Intimate Relationship

__ Quality of Sleep

__ Overall health

In which area are you the least satisfied?

_____

What action step do you want to take to raise your satisfaction?

_____

In which area are you the most satisfied?

In which area are you the next most satisfied?

_____

How could you increase your level of satisfaction in this level even further?

_____

Make a list of the things you are grateful for and meditate on these.

_____

_____

_____

_____

_____

_____

_____

_____

_____

Step 7: It's the Thought That Counts

You've heard it said that "thoughts are things".

Dr. Candace Pert, in her book, *The Molecules of Emotion*, discovered that thoughts actually have chemicals attached to them that travel throughout the body, affecting our immune systems and our organs.

As you might guess, negative thoughts have negative effects and positive thoughts have positive effects. So, is the answer simply to think positive thoughts?

We've all been encouraged to think more positively, do affirmations, etc. But maybe it's not that easy. Maybe you don't get the privilege of selecting your thoughts. Maybe your thoughts come unbidden, like intruders in the night.

Research has shown that most of us have between 12,000 and 60,000 thoughts a day, and of these, a large percentage are the same thoughts we had the day before. Sound familiar?

However, even though you don't select your thoughts, you do get to select which thoughts you choose to dwell on.

If positive thoughts have positive physiological payoffs, then why not deliberately nurture these rather than endlessly obsessing over the negative ones? After all, you do have a choice!

Before you can banish a negative thought, you need to become aware that you are having it. You have to catch it before you can eliminate it.

You can do this by monitoring your feelings. Thoughts create feelings. If you're feeling unhappy, stop to recollect your last thoughts. These are your triggers. Your previous thoughts have created the present feelings. So, start by identifying those thoughts.

Now, you have a choice, Replace the negative thought with something more positive, or deal with the thoughts so that you reach resolution and can put it to rest. This may be something you can do alone, or you may need the help of a trusted confidante, therapist, or coach to help you reframe the troubling thought into something more uplifting.

This may not be easily accomplished but it's definitely do-able. For example, if you are obsessing over a particular worry, allow your mind to go to the worst case scenario.

Your mind is going to go there anyway, so you might as well take charge of the process.

Then make a plan as to how you'll handle it if the worst occurs. Just the act of making the plan is calming and reassuring. Things don't go nearly as awry as people anticipate. So much worry is needless suffering. Thoughts are like wild horses, and need a rider to take the reins. Take the reins. Take charge of your thoughts!

In fact, guard your thoughts like the gold in Fort Knox, because positive thoughts are worth their weight in gold!

The Skinny

Now that you know your numbers and understand how your habits and emotions affect your risk of developing diabetes, let's summarize some of the new behaviors that you can incorporate for weight loss and better health.

Your body needs a combination of protein, carbohydrates, and fats. It's important to eat the right kinds of proteins, carbohydrates, and fats, and to eat them in appropriate portion sizes with each meal.

New guidelines suggest that half of your plate should consist of fruits and vegetables, and the other half consist of proteins, carbohydrates, and a small portion of fats.

It usually takes around 20 minutes for your brain to get the message that you're full. How much food can you eat in 20 minutes? If you're a fast eater, quite a lot!

The key here is to slow down. If you pay attention to every bite, you're much more likely to feel satisfied with less food in your stomach.

One of the worst distractions while eating is the TV. When you watch TV, you're lulled into a TV trance. If you don't think so, just recall the many times that you knew you should turn off the set, but continued to stare at the screen. Watching television is hypnotic. How many times have you sat through commercials on programs that you taped? You were in a trance, my friend. And when you eat in front of the TV, you eat mindlessly, and many times, too quickly.

Sometimes you have to a limited time to eat. I used to be the slowest eater at the table until I became a teacher. With 25 minutes to get through the lunch line and eat, I had to speed it up or go hungry. This is a recipe for indigestion and weight gain. I had to re-train myself to slow down and eat mindfully.

Ask yourself how to best slow down your eating. Slow and steady wins the race...the race to health, that is!

Now let's talk about portion control. The "all you can eat" philosophy not going to cut it. Use smaller plates to make your servings appear larger.

The name of the game is change. You need to reduce your portions to reduce your calories.

This doesn't have to be a drastic change. Small changes can produce big results.

Fruits, vegetables, nuts, and lean meats are all low glycemic and nutritional without spiking your blood sugar. If you stick to these foods, avoid white foods, sodas, and sugars, you'll keep your blood sugar steady and you won't suffer from cravings.

Adding fiber to your menu also keeps your blood sugar from spiking. It slows down the entire operation.

If you eat every 3 or 4 hours, you'll keep yourself from becoming hungry.

If you drink enough water throughout the day, your body won't mistake dehydration for hunger.

If you add a little exercise to your daily routine, you won't feel as hungry and you'll be more likely to eat healthy foods.

Finally, if you begin to practice healthy, low glycemic eating, you'll lose weight without even trying. And when you lose weight, your risk for diabetes goes down. And isn't that the point?

If this seems like a daunting task, incorporate one new behavior a week. Before you know it, you'll have a healthy new lifestyle and the body you desire!

It's your life. You deserve good health. Many times, hiring a coach to support you, guide you, and keep you accountable for making the changes you want to make, can greatly increase your chances for success. Weight loss can be a challenging task to attempt alone.

Whether you decide to achieve this goal alone or with the support of a coach, good health is your birth right. After all, how long do you want to live? Whatever the number, you can follow your roadmap to peace, health, and happiness. It's your life…

Go for it!

About the Author

Teresa Trower M.A. LMHC. is a Licensed Mental Health Counselor and "Baby Boomer Weight Loss Coach" in Jacksonville Florida.

As a former teacher and Guidance Counselor, Teresa has authored several publications for children, including *Furious Fables, Self Esteem Stories, The Self Control Patrol* (a board game), *and the Self Control Patrol Workbook.*

In her private practice, Teresa helps clients avoid a diagnosis of Type 2 Diabetes through her "Weight Loss and Stress Resilience" coaching program. This program also includes smoking cessation, weight loss hypnosis, and Life Purpose and Self Love coaching.

Her CD, *Hypnosis Meditation for Weight Loss,* is available on her website.

For more information about Teresa and her programs, please visit the following websites:

www.stressbustercoach.com

www.tenpoundslost.com

Bibliography:

Alzheimer's Disease Could Be A Third Form of Diabetes. Science Daily. Sept. 27, 2007

Anastassios G. Pittas, MD, MSc, Joseph Lau, MD, Frank HU, MD, Bess Dawson-Hughes, MD. The Role of Vitamin D and Calcium in type 2 Diabetes: A Systematic Review andMeta-Analysis. http://www.ncbi.nlm.nih.gov/pmc/articles/PMC2085234/

Causes of Type 2 Diabetes. Diabetes Health Center. http://diabetes.webmd.com/guide/diabetes-causes, June 25, 2011

Chang, Julie, Seshamani, MD, Phd, Department of Health and Human Services. Preventing and Treating Diabetes: Health Insurance Reform and Diabetes in America http://advocacy.diabetes.org/site/DocServer/HHS_Diabetes_Health_Reform_report.pdf?docID=33841

Davidson, Jaleh. Tips for Curbing Your Craving for Sweets and Carbs: Interview with Teresa Trower, M.A. LMHC. http://www.associatedcontent.com/article/7752418/tips_for_curbing_your_craving_for_sweets.html?cat=5Feb 24, 2011

Diabetes and Medicare: One Patient's Story.
Health.com. c2010

Does Emotional Stress Cause Type 2 Diabetes
Mellitus? A Review from the European Depression
in Diabetes Research Consortium

FAWCO. New cholesterol testing.
http://www.fawco.org/index.php?option=com_co
ntent&view=article&id=312:new-cholesterol-
testing&catid=109:health-issues&Itemid=100563

Florida Times Union. An Apple A Day, Smarty
Pants.Health and Fitness. July 20, 2011

Glenn, Stephen. Developing Capable Young People.
http://www.capabilitiesinc.com/glenn.html

Good vs. Bad Cholesterol. American Heart
Association.
http://www.heart.org/HEARTORG/Conditions/
Cholesterol/AboutCholesterol/Good-vs-Bad-
Cholesterol_UCM_305561_Article.jsp, June, 2011

Haiken, Melanie. 5 Foods That Can Trigger a Stroke.
Yahoo!Health. http://health.yahoo.net/caring/5-
foods-that-can-trigger-a-stroke

High Glycemic Foods. HealthAliciousness.com
http://www.healthaliciousness.com/blog/List-
Common-High-Glycemic-Index-GI-foods-which-
can-be-eliminated.php

How To Prevent Pre- Diabetes. American Diabetes Association. http://www.diabetes.org/diabetes-basics/prevention/pre-diabetes/how-to-prevent-pre-diabetes.html

Hyman, Dr. Mark. Is Your Body Burning Up With Hidden Inflammation? www.drhyman.com/topic/inflammation.

Nauert ,Rick, PhD, Stress Hormone Affects Immune System. Psychcentral.com. 2008

Patterson, Kerry, Grenny, Joseph, Maxfield, David, McMillan, Ron, Switzler, al. Change Anything. http://www.amazon.com/Change-Anything-Science-Personal-Success/dp/0446573914

Pert, Candace, PhD. Molecules of Emotion. http://books.simonandschuster.ca/Molecules-of-Emotion/Candace-B-Pert-Ph-D/9780743541398

Pick, Marcelle, OB/GYN NP. Reducing Inflammation, the Natural Approach. http://www.womentowomen.com/inflammation/naturalantiinflammatories.aspx, April 20, 2011

Roan, Sheri. Anxiety Disorders May Precede Diabetes in Latinos. Los Angeles Times. http://www.latimes.com/health/boostershots/la-heb-latino-diabetes-20110520,0,7940327.story, May 20, 201

Ross, Healther M. The Dangers of High Cholesterol and. Diabetes.
http://cholesterol.about.com/lw/Health-Medicine/Conditions-and-diseases/The-Dangers-of-High-Cholesterol-If-You-Have-Diabetes.htm, Oct.2010

Shoman, Mary. What is the Optimal TSH Level for Thyroid Patients?
http://thyroid.about.com/od/gettestedanddiagnosed/a/optimaltsh.htm, Sept. 14, 2006

Strand, Dr. Ray D, MD. Healthy for Life. Real Life Press, 2005.

Understanding Cholesterol Numbers. Cholesterol Management Health Center.
http://www.webmd.com/cholesterol-management/guide/understanding-numbers, June 25, 2011

Wolfe, Dr. Karen. Glycemic Stress. Webinar. Usana Health Science. 2011.

Notes:

www.ingramcontent.com/pod-product-compliance
Lightning Source LLC
Chambersburg PA
CBHW070200290526
45789CB00002B/854